Mighty - Me and the Rainbow Plate

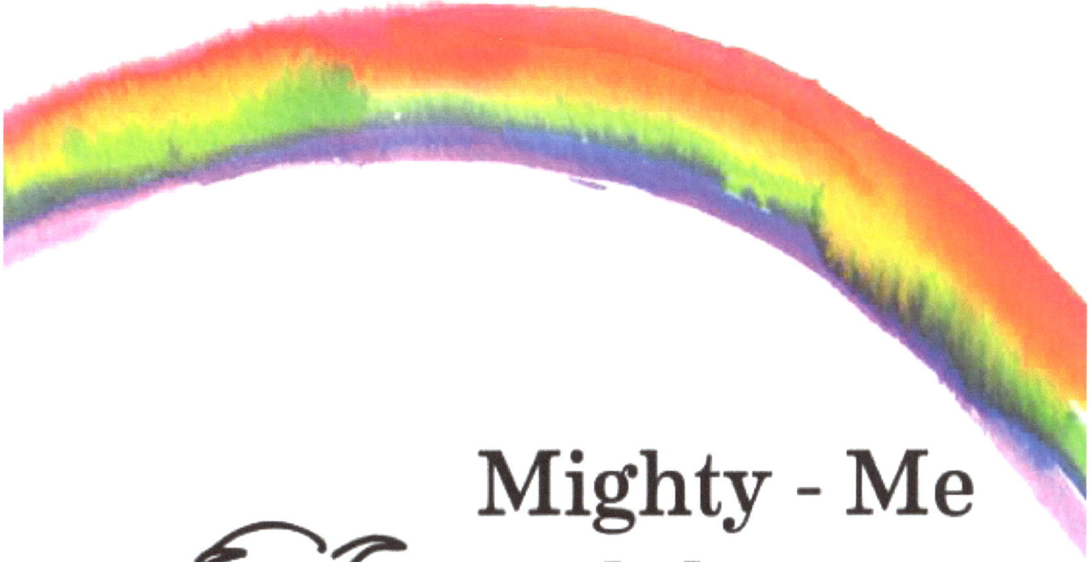

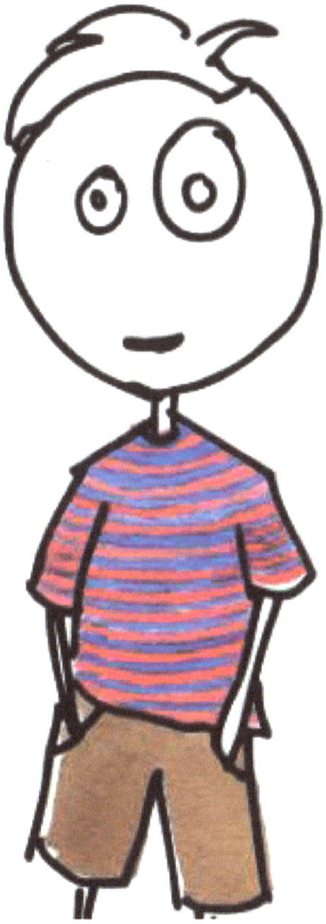

Margery Phelps

Illustrations By Julie Weinberger

Apple Pie Books - Atlanta, GA

Mighty-Me and the Rainbow Plate

ISB N
13: 978-1479196616
10: 1479196614

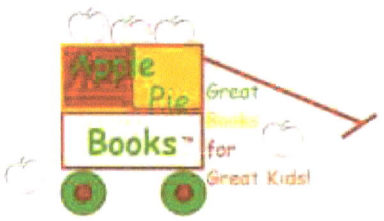

www.ApplePieBooks.com

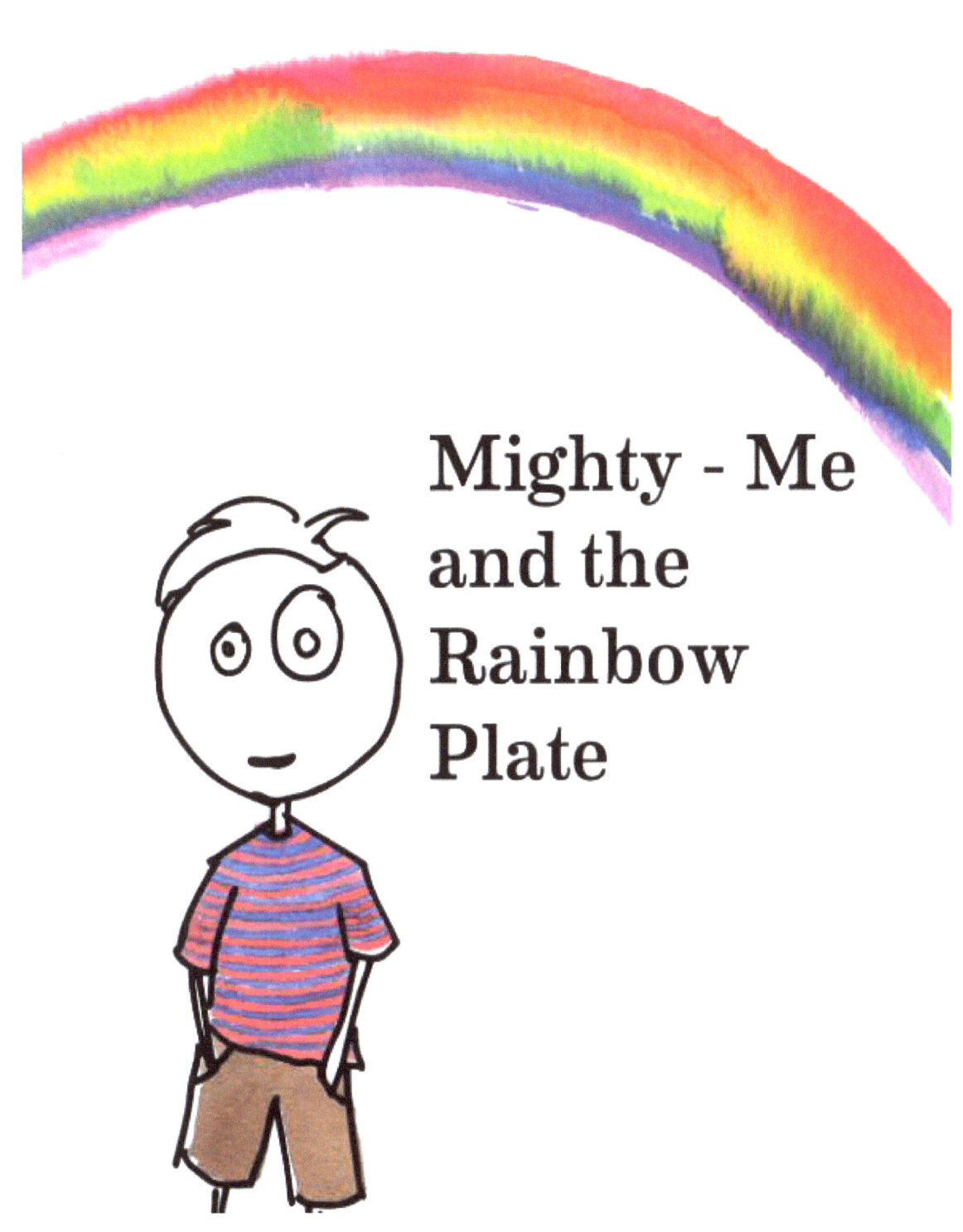

Mighty - Me and the Rainbow Plate

There was a Kid, not very big
who did not like to eat...

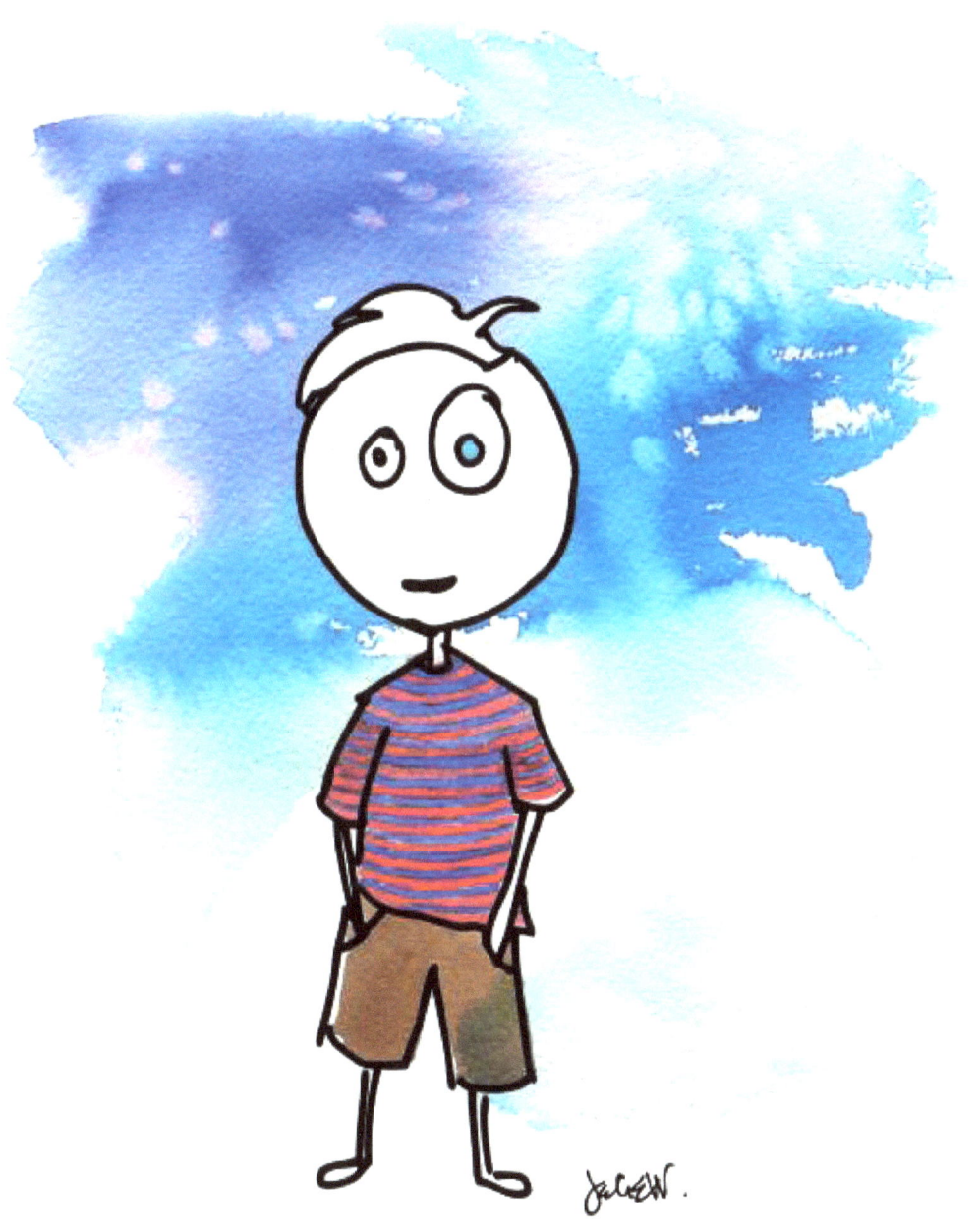

...the things that would be good for Kids
like fruits and vegetables and meat.

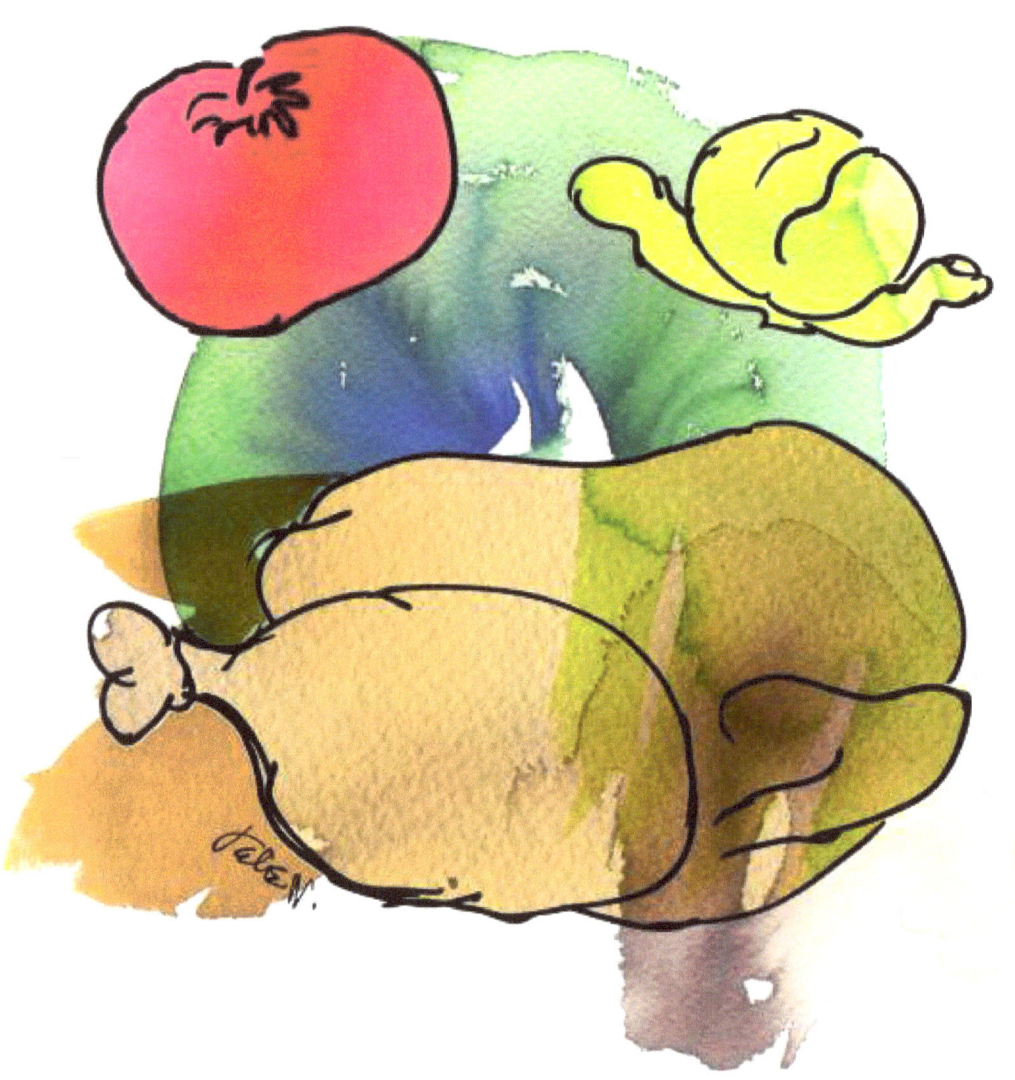

But, oh, did Kid like French fries,
and great big cola drinks.

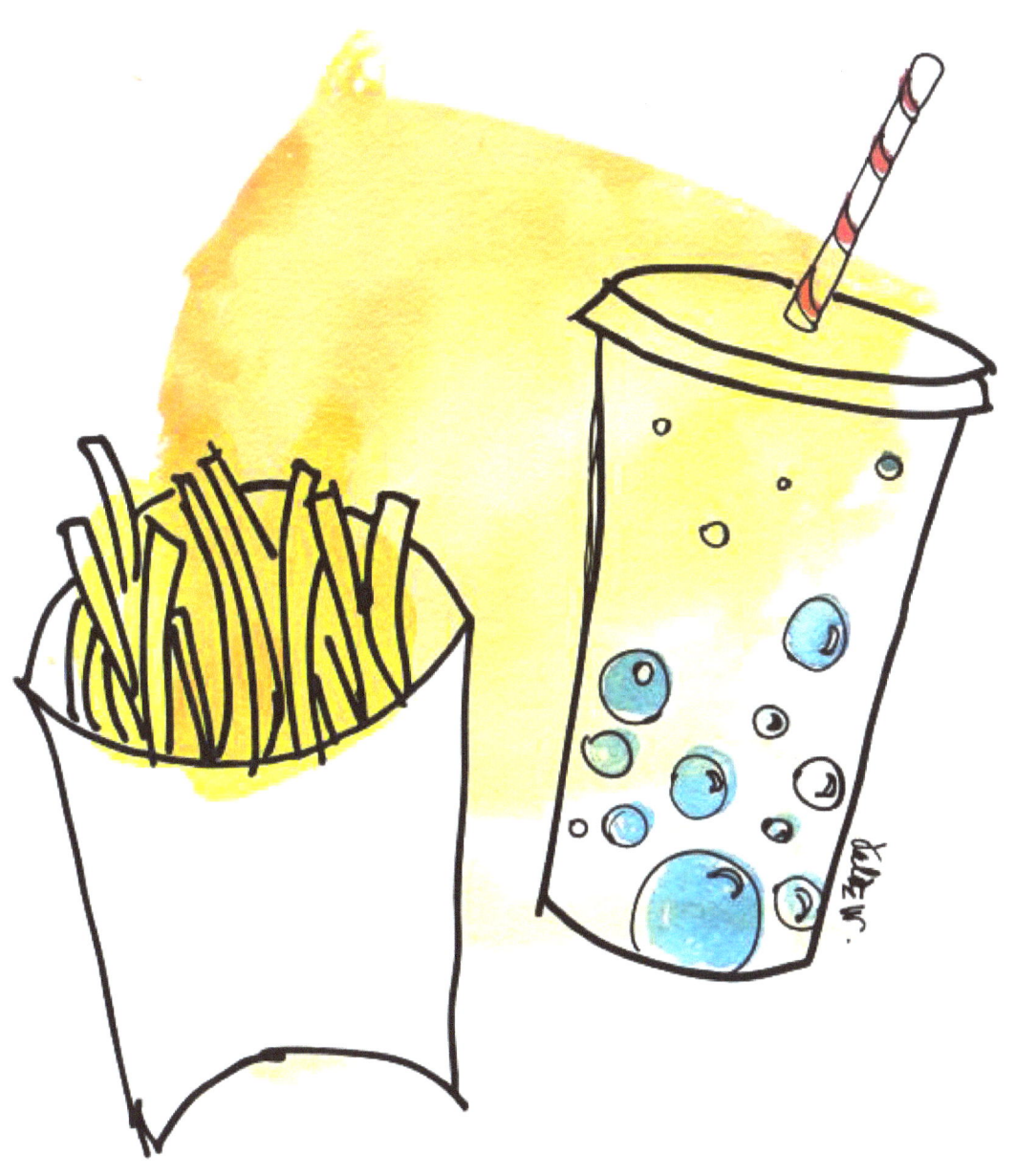

And oh my goodness those pizza pies,
would be eaten as quick as a wink.

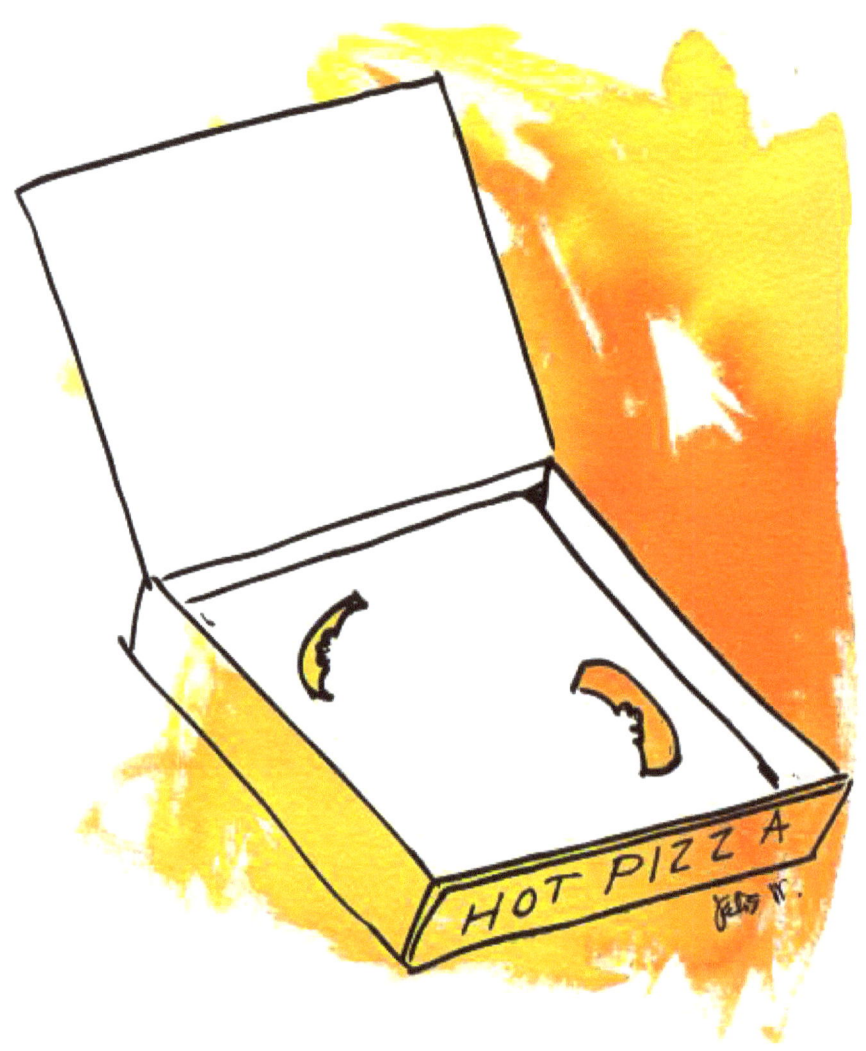

Then Kid got bigger and went to school,

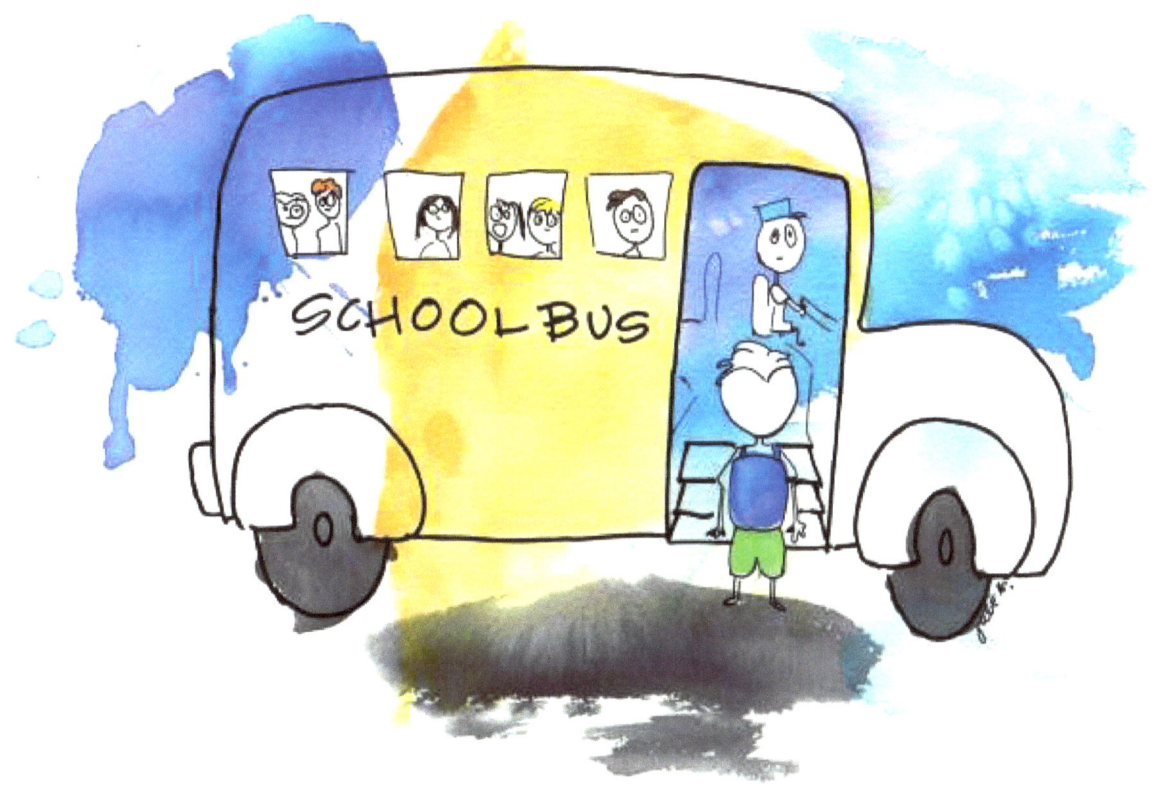

and rode upon the bus.

Because Kid knew the Golden Rule
he did not fight or fuss.

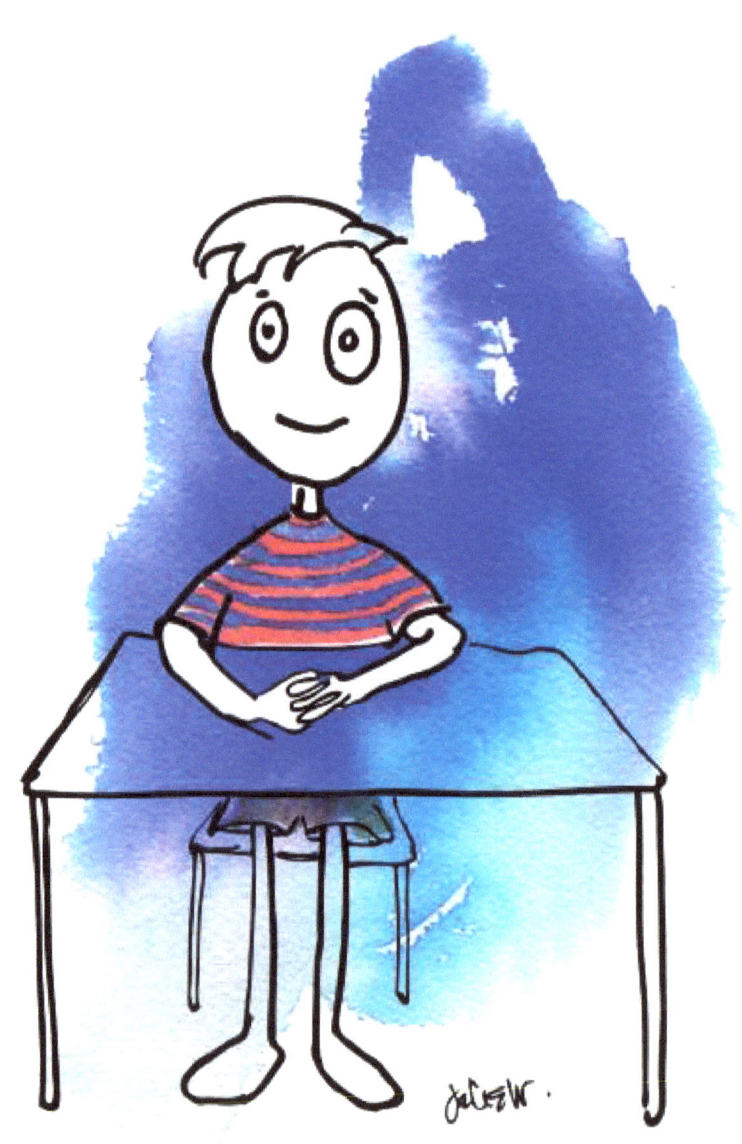

The teacher was so very nice,

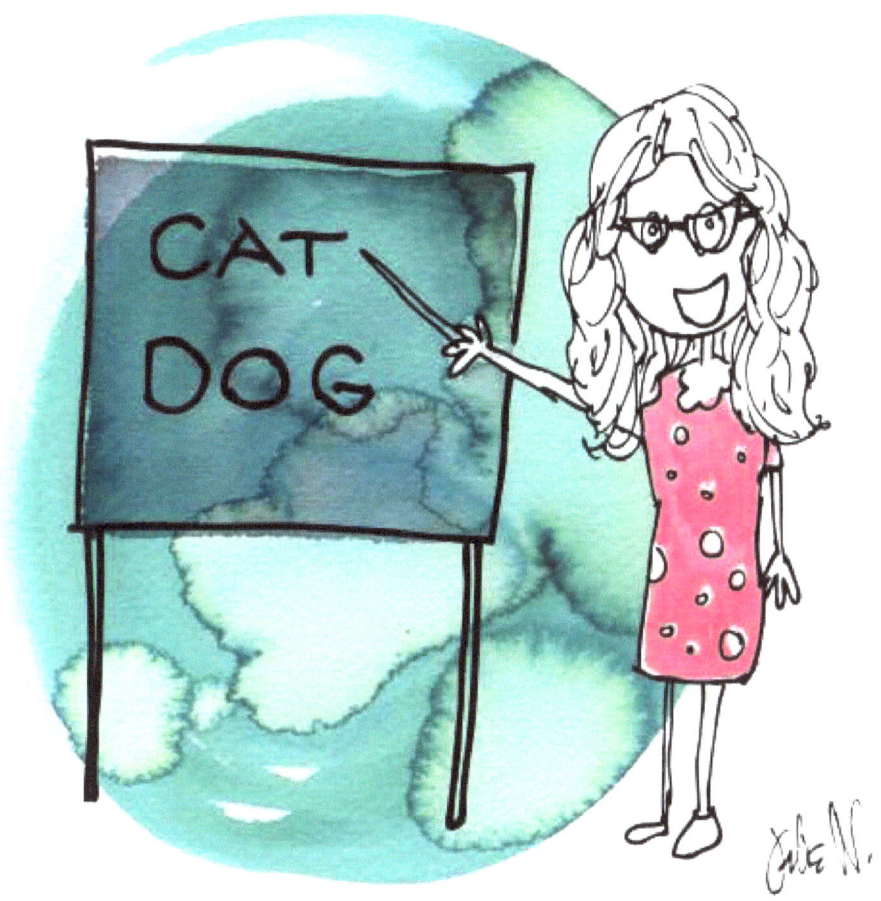

she taught the kids to read and write.

And how to be a quiet as mice - -

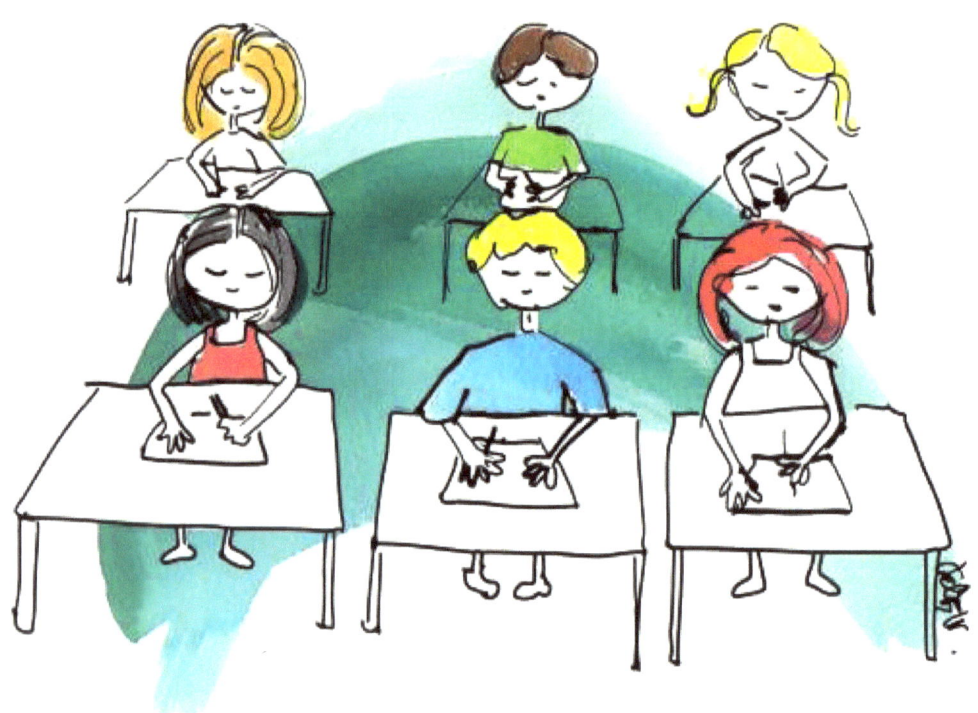

everyone in class was so polite.

They learned to write their A - B - Cs
and how to count their numbers.

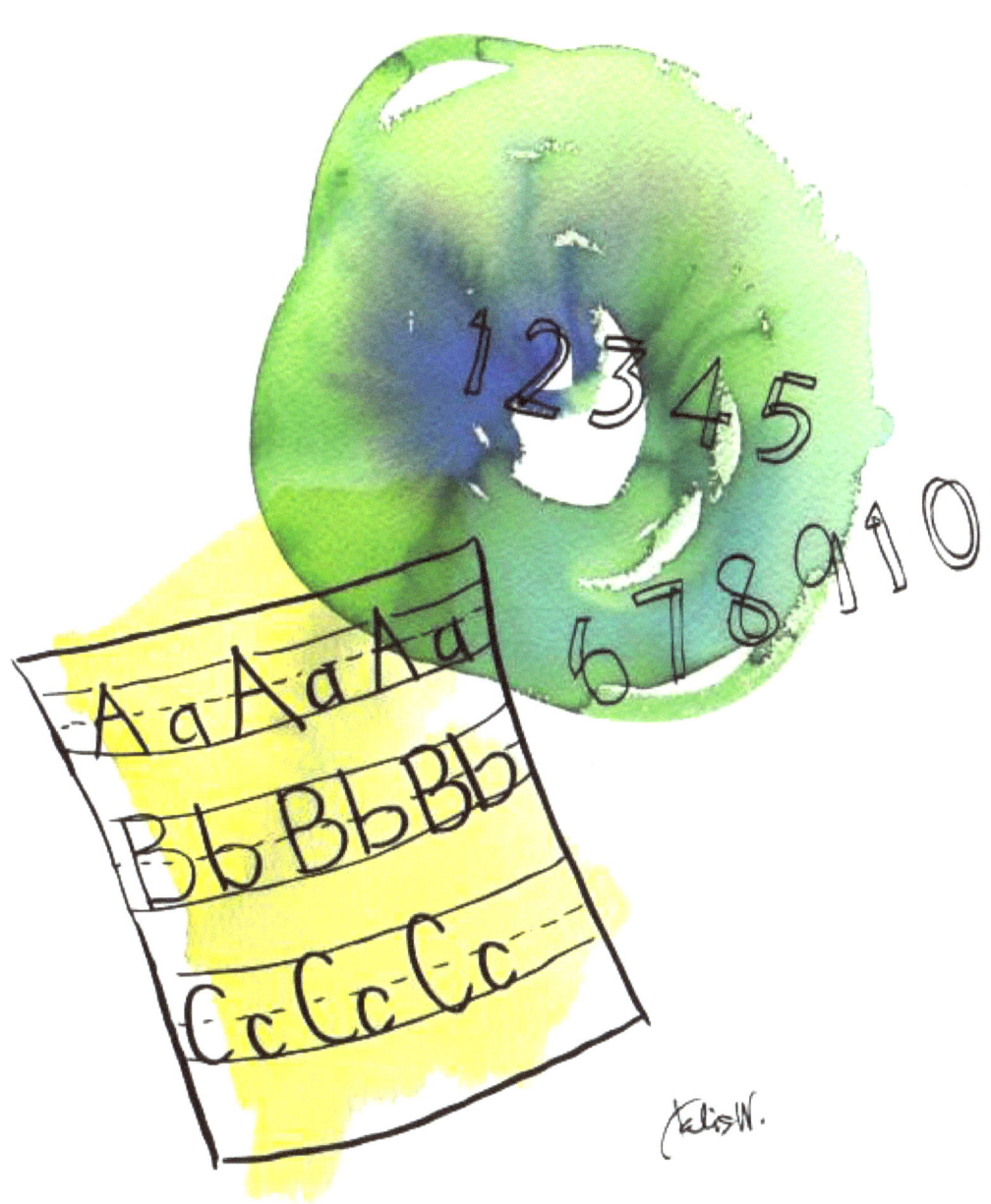

School was fun, as fun can be,
it was full of marvelous wonders.

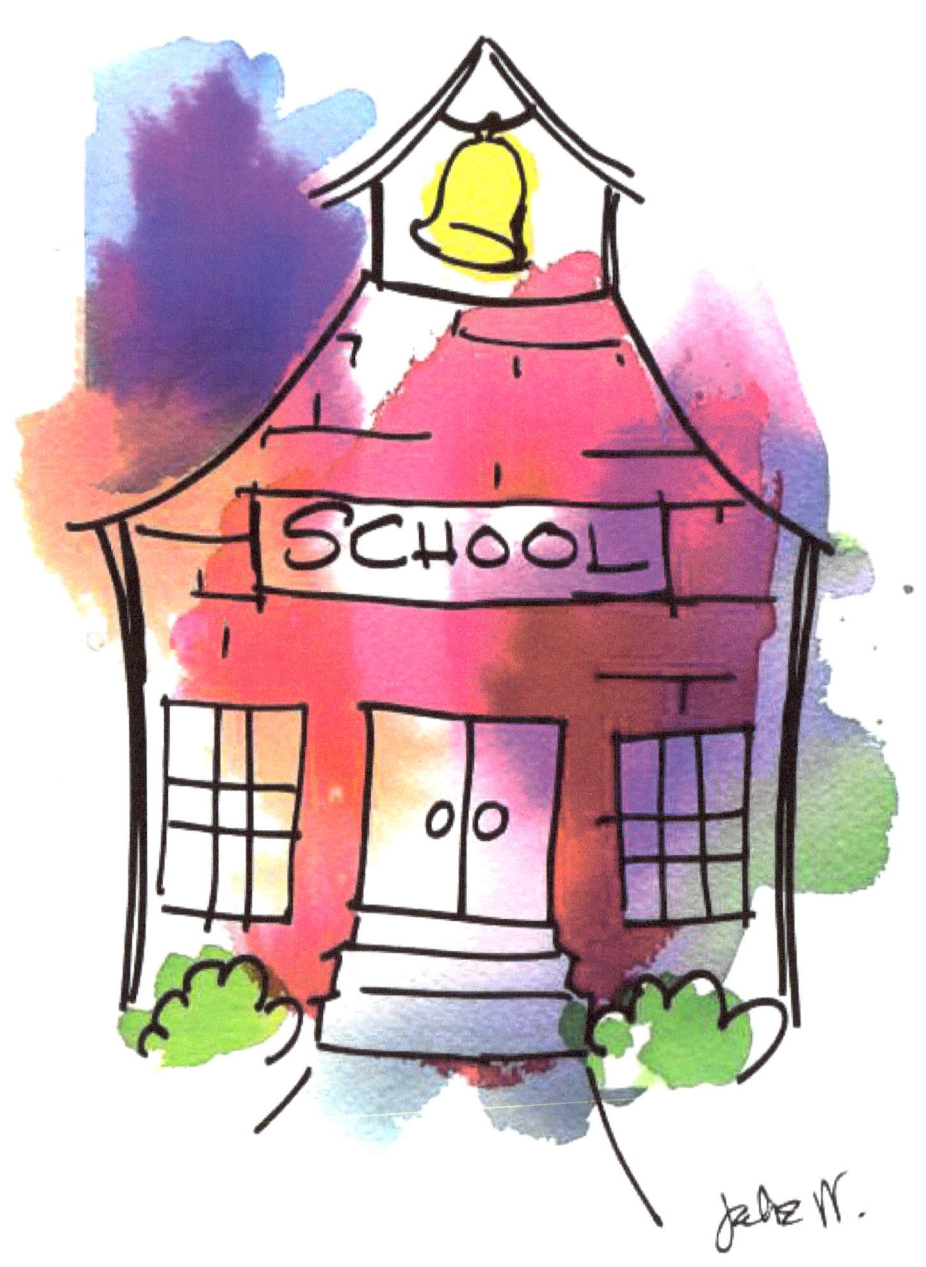

At lunch time they were ready to eat,

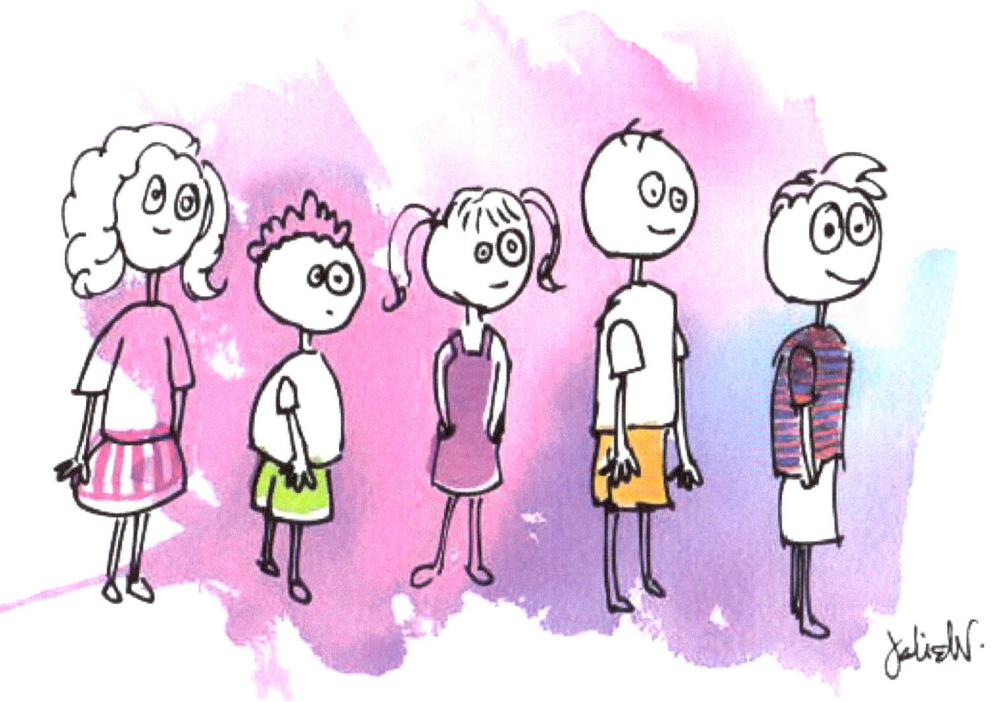

so the Kids got in a line.

And went to the cafeteria,

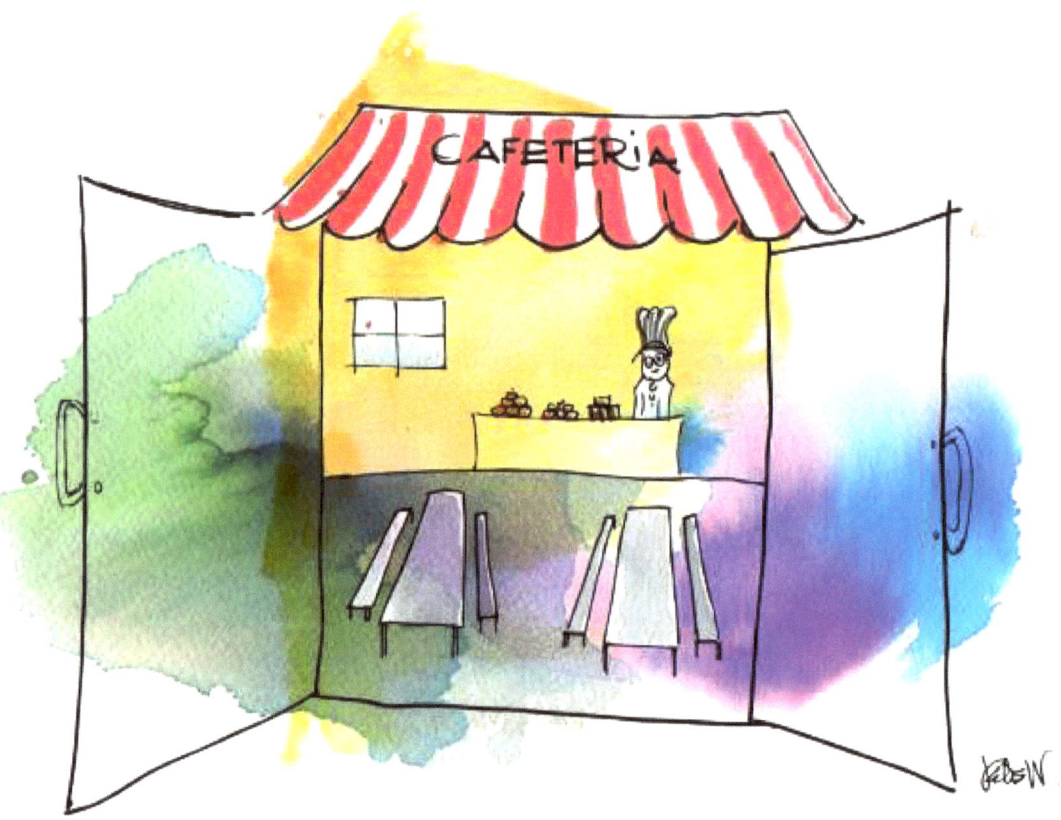

where the food was really fine.

12

The cafeteria at the fantastic school
served fruits and vegetables and meat.

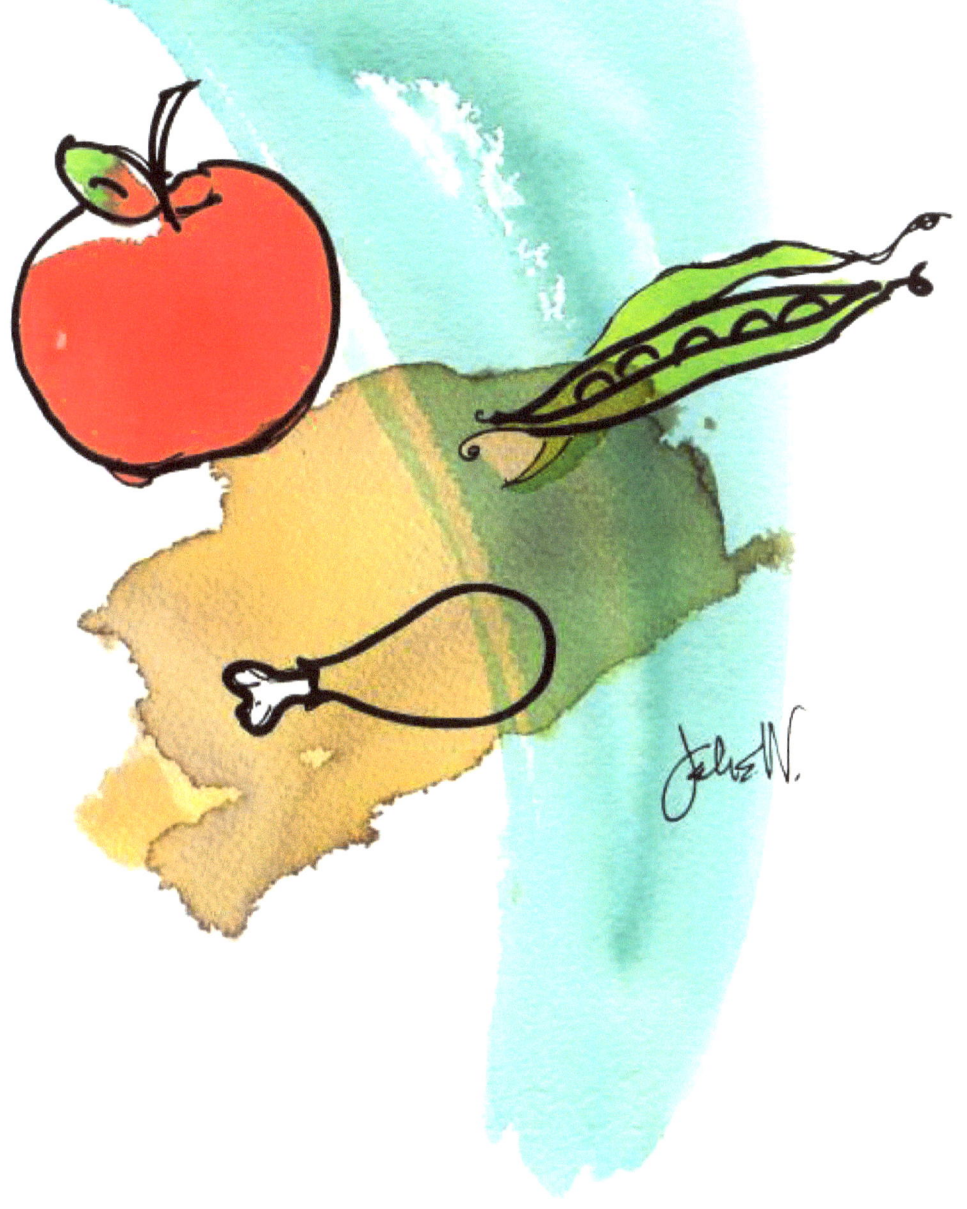

But the kids all thought that it was cool

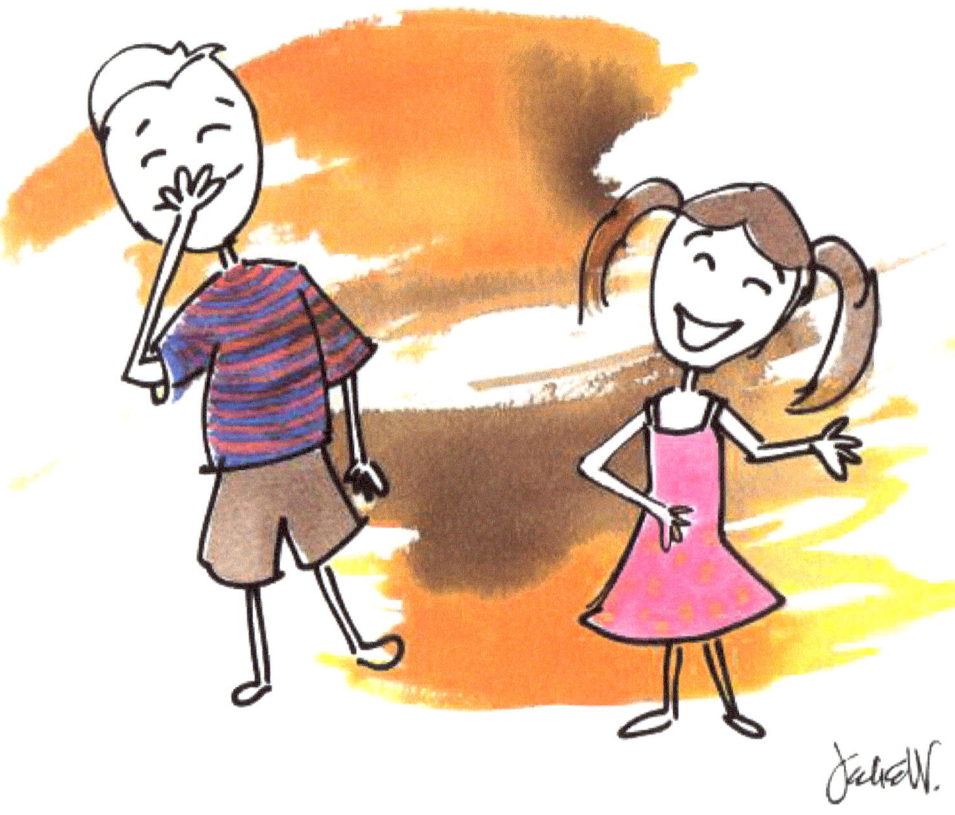

to make fun of the food they would not eat.

After lunch, the kids were kind of
sleepy

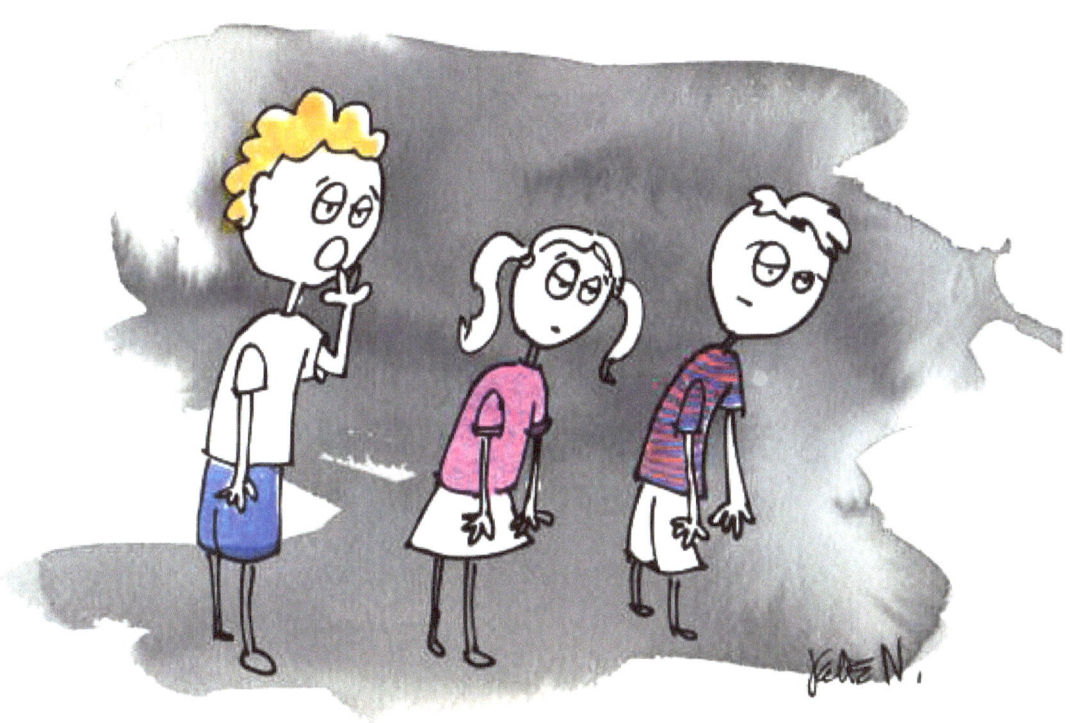

'cause they hardly ate a bite.

They didn't want to play outside,

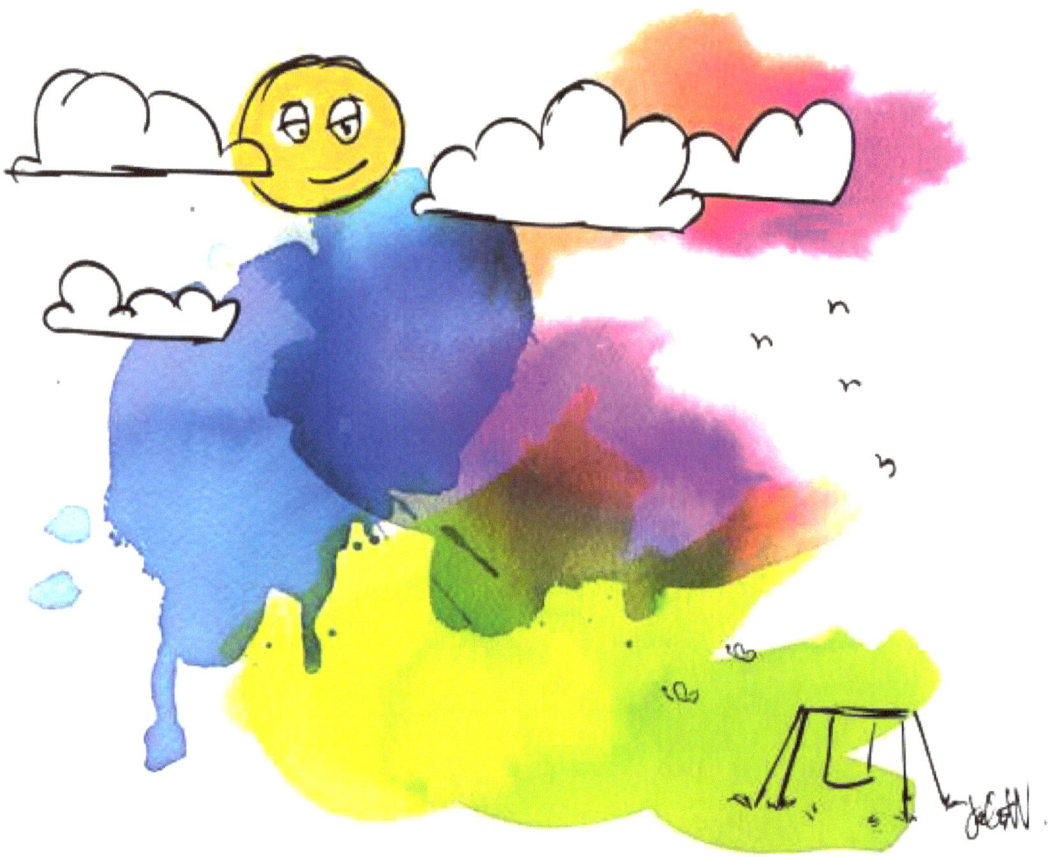

where the sun was shining bright.

And they got really, really grumpy,
and almost started a fight.

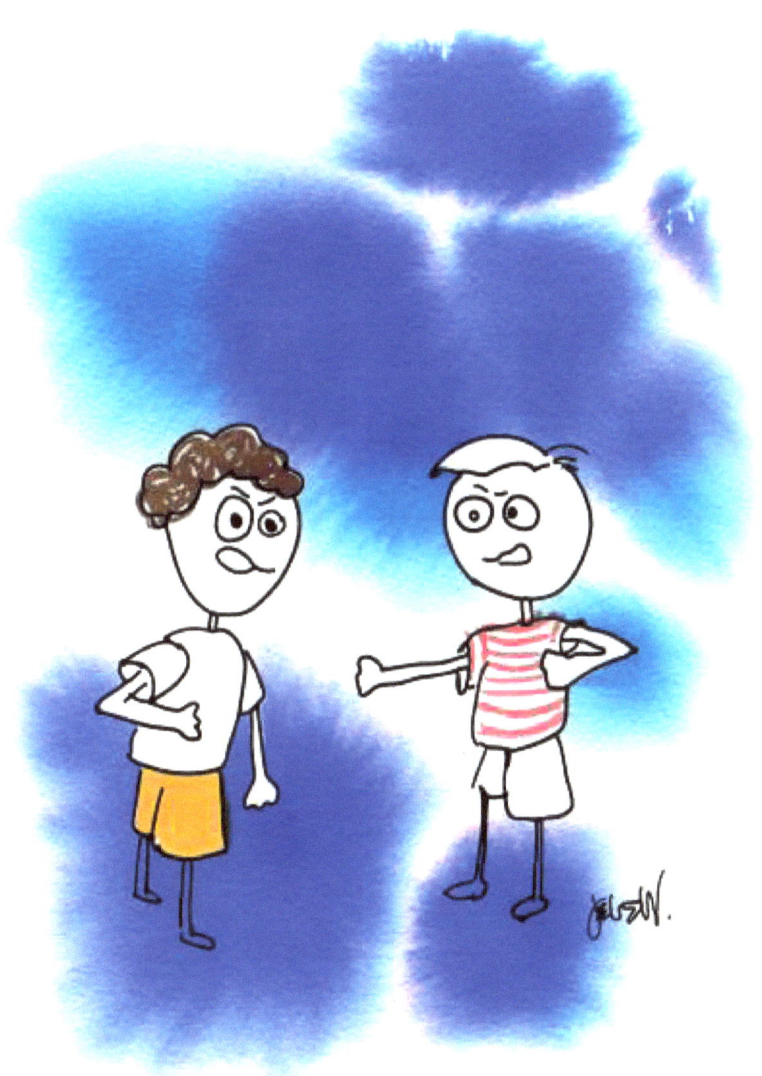

Then Teacher said,
"Let's get this straight,

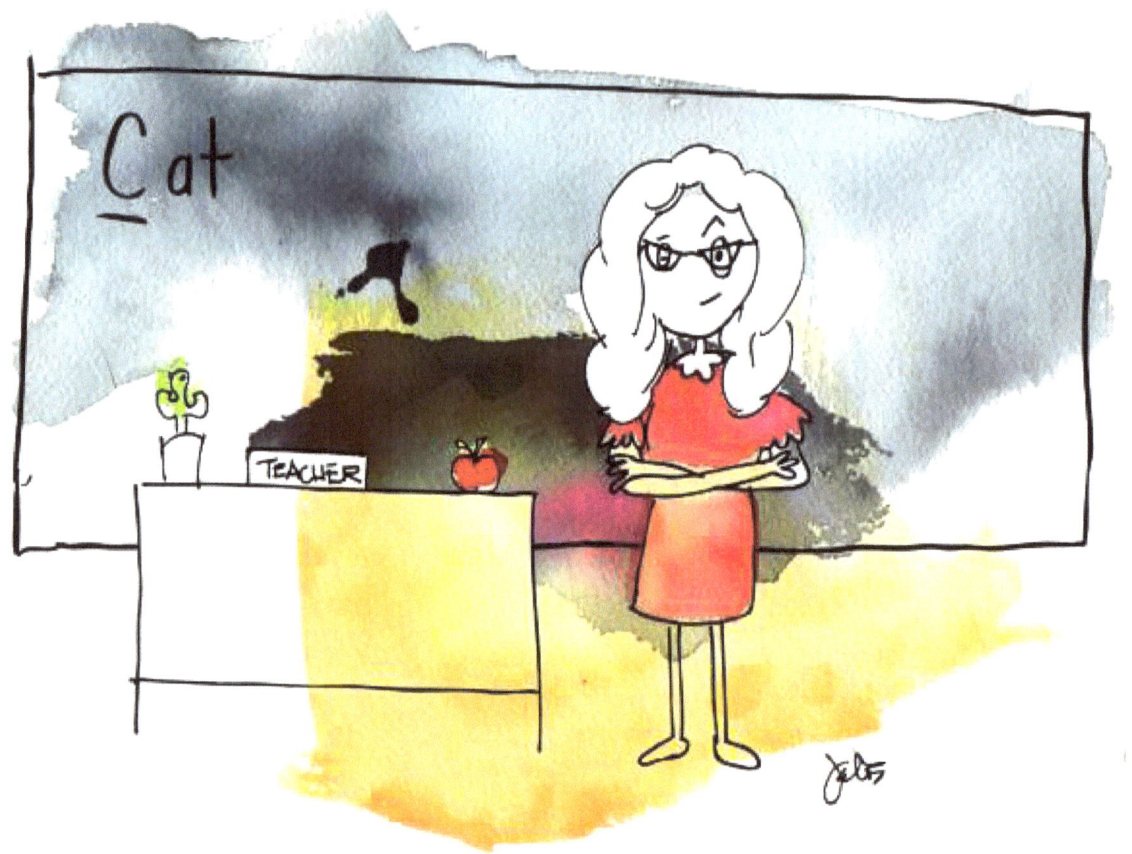

You say you're too tired to play!"

"If you had eaten what's on your plate,

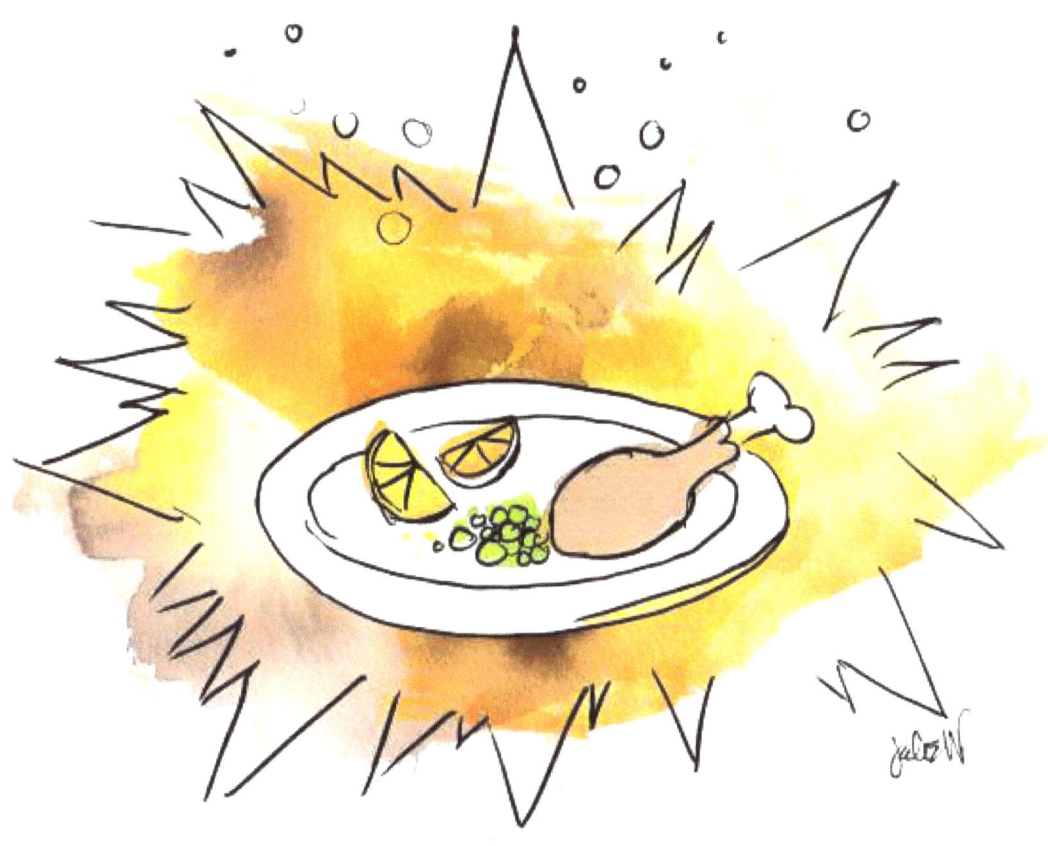

you'd have the energy to play all day."

It started to rain,
and the thunder roared.

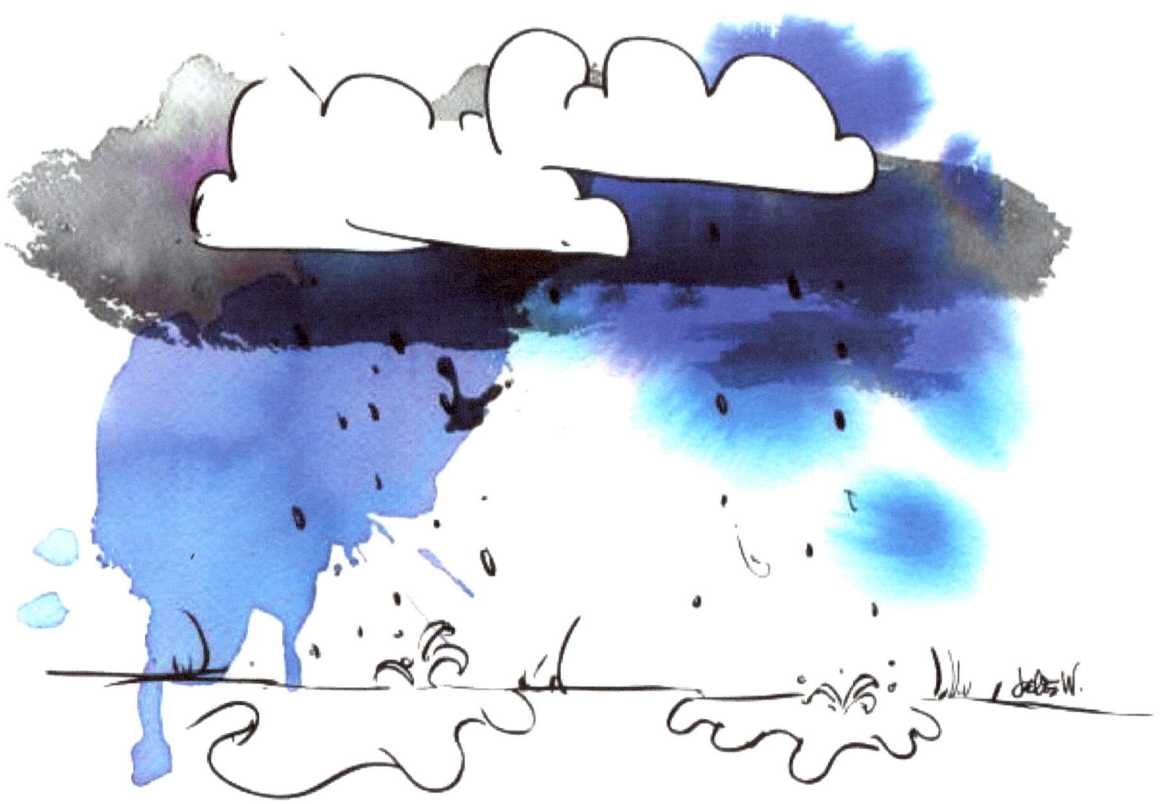

It gave them all a terrible fright.

When the storm was over
above them soared

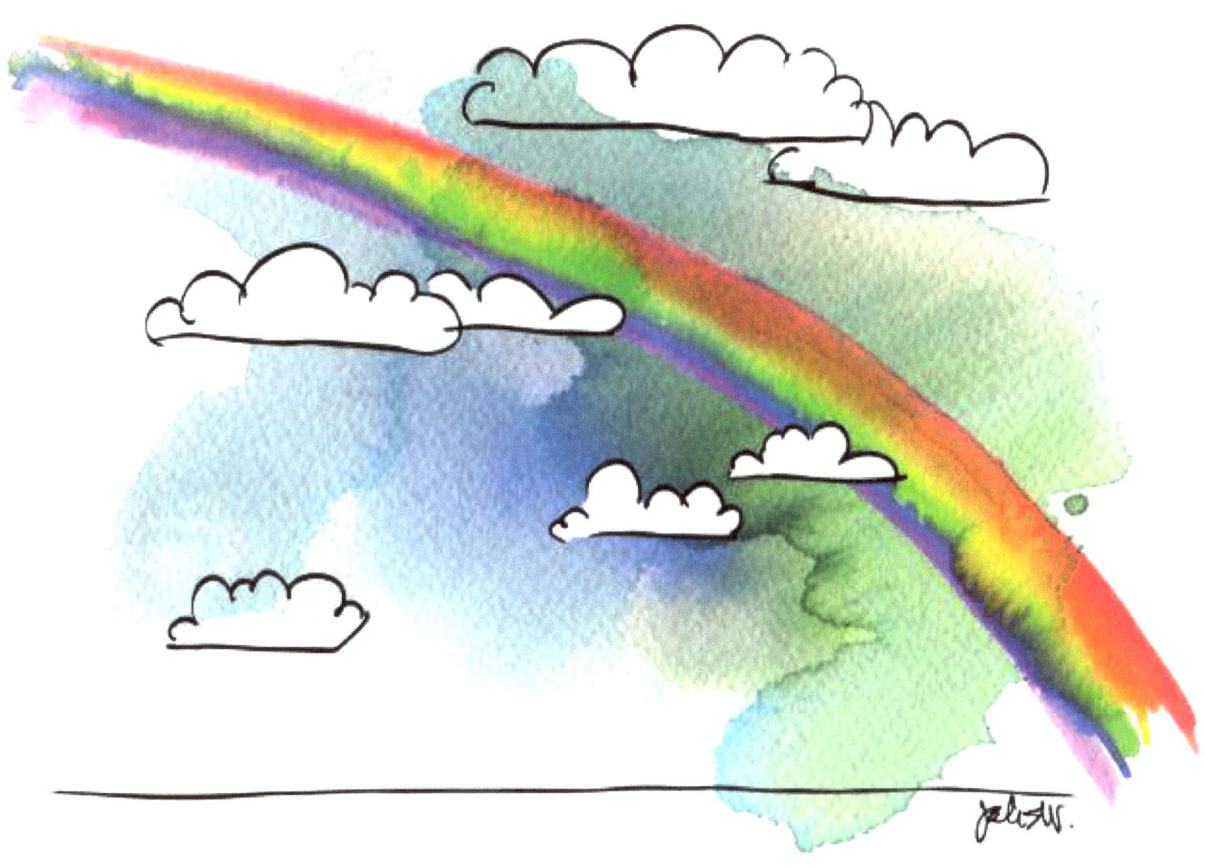

a rainbow with colors so bright.

"What do all those colors mean?"
  the children wanted to know.

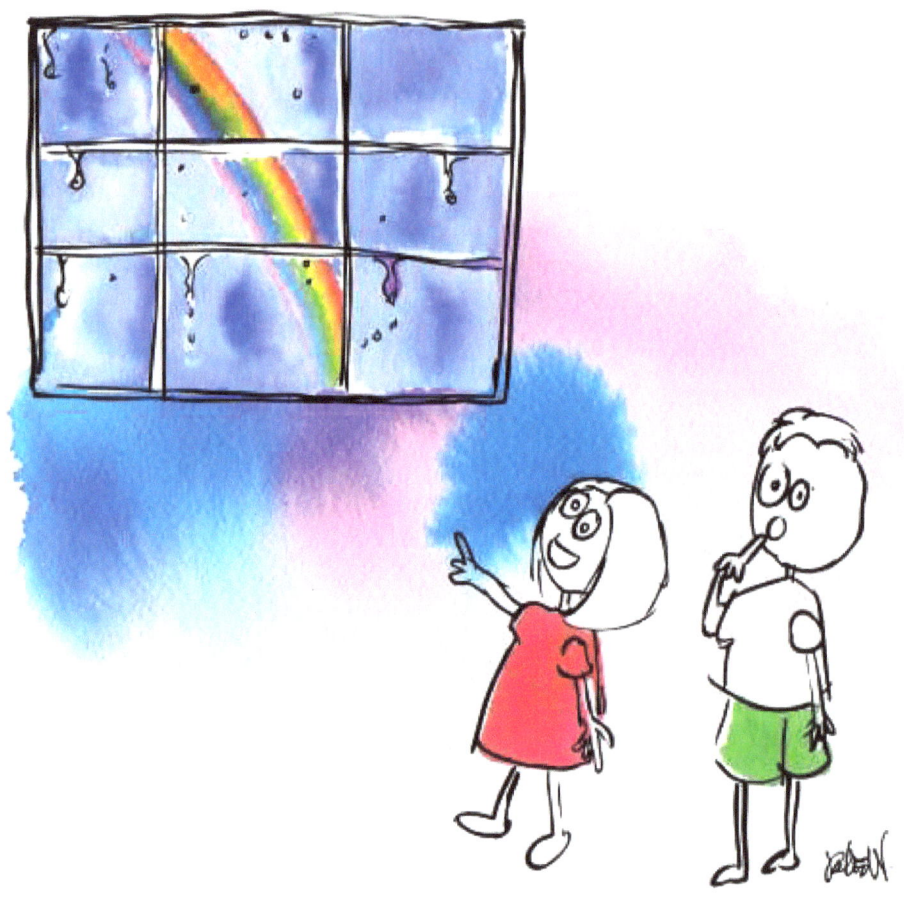

"Why is there red and yellow and green?
  Why is the sky all aglow?"

22

"Well think about it,"
the teacher said

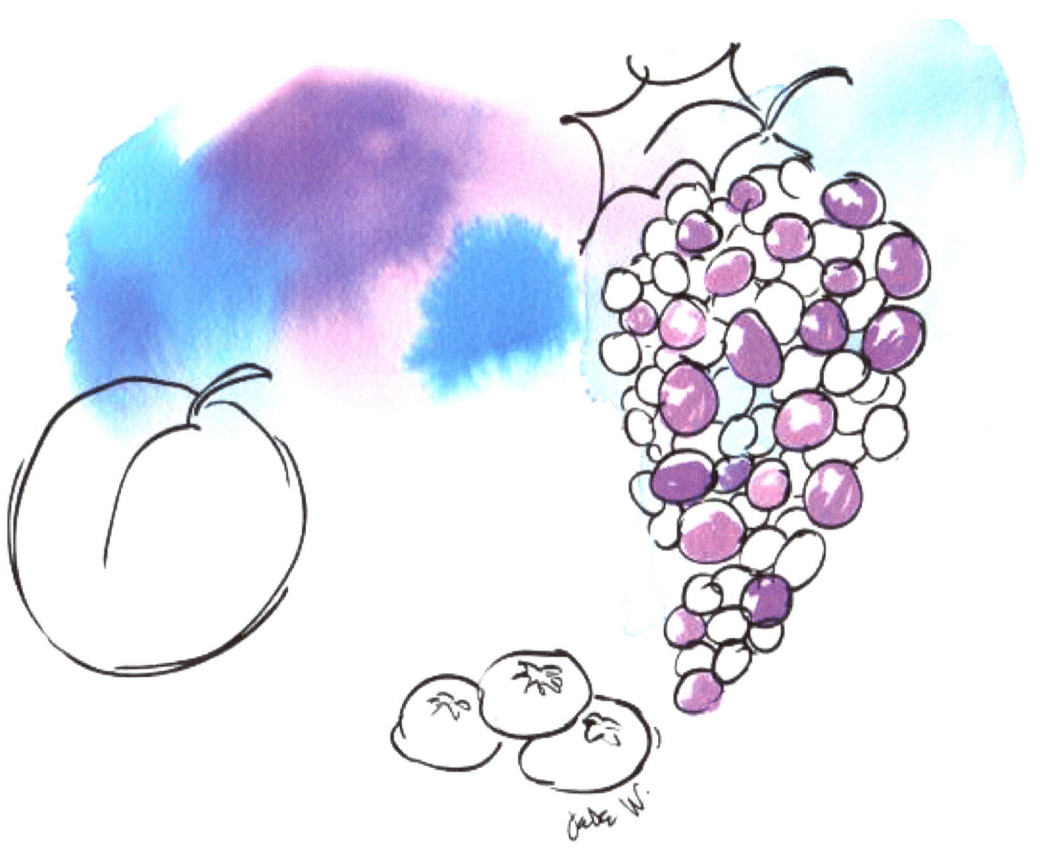

"What do you eat that's purple or blue?"

"And what do you eat that's
really bright red?

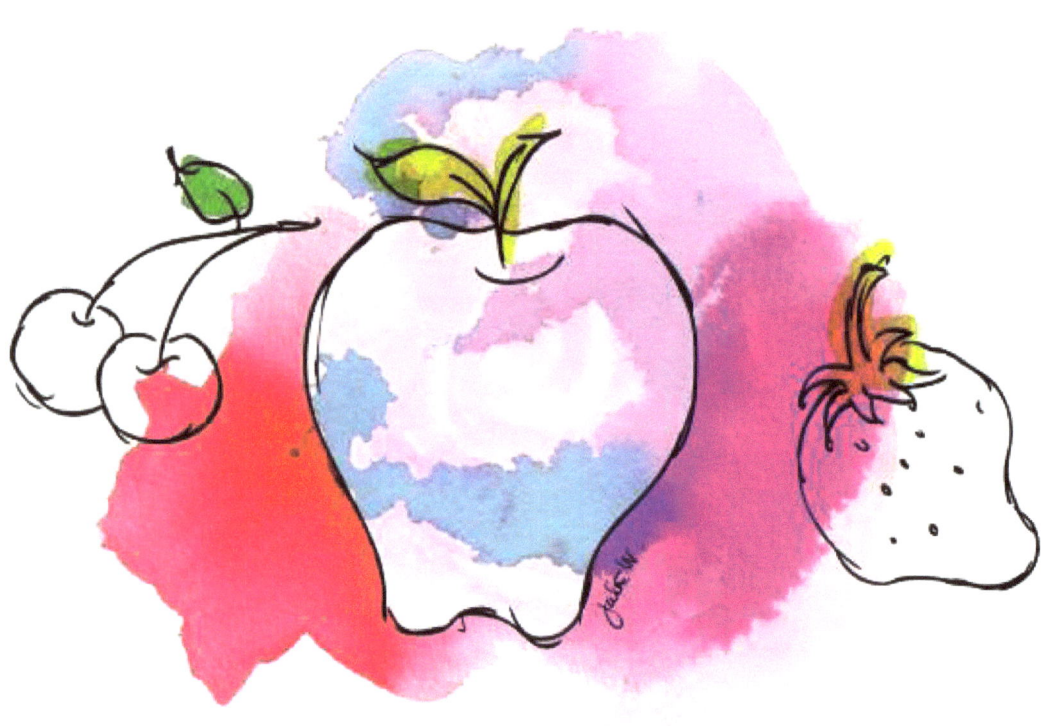

Oh, I forgot,
you won't eat food that's good for you."

24

"You mean the Rainbow in the sky
is the color of things
we should eat and drink?

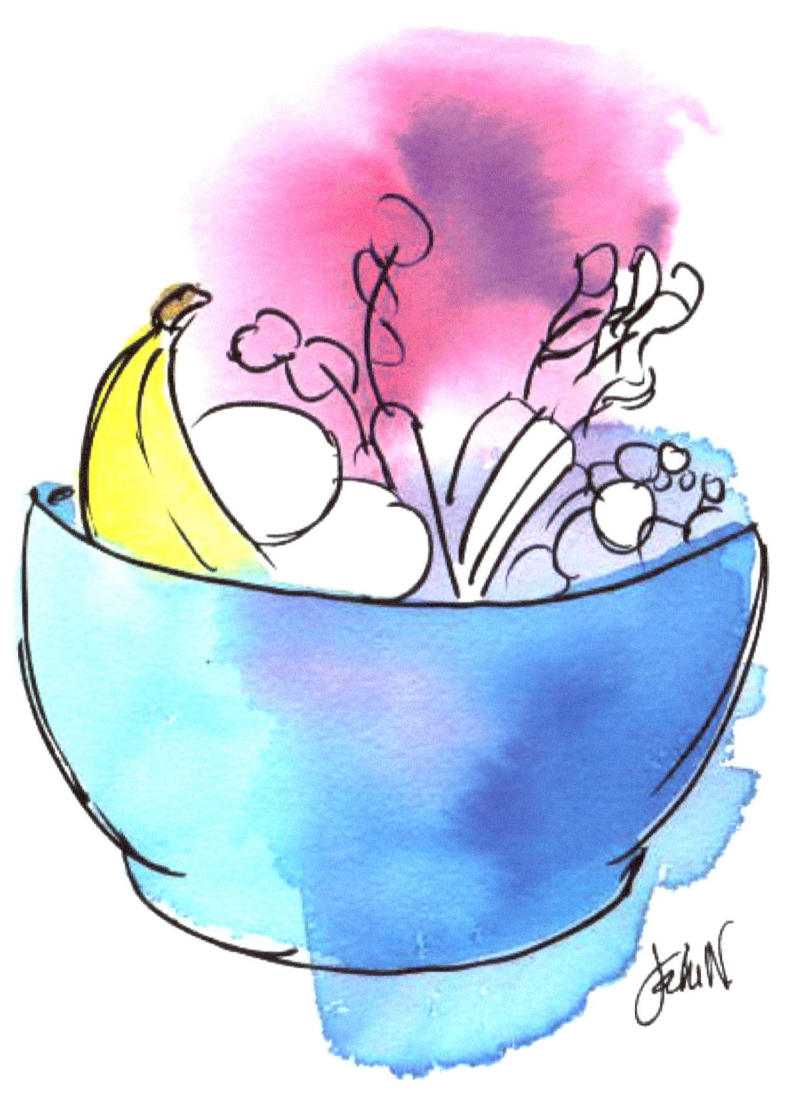

"By all means," Teacher did reply,
And she gave the Kids a great big wink.

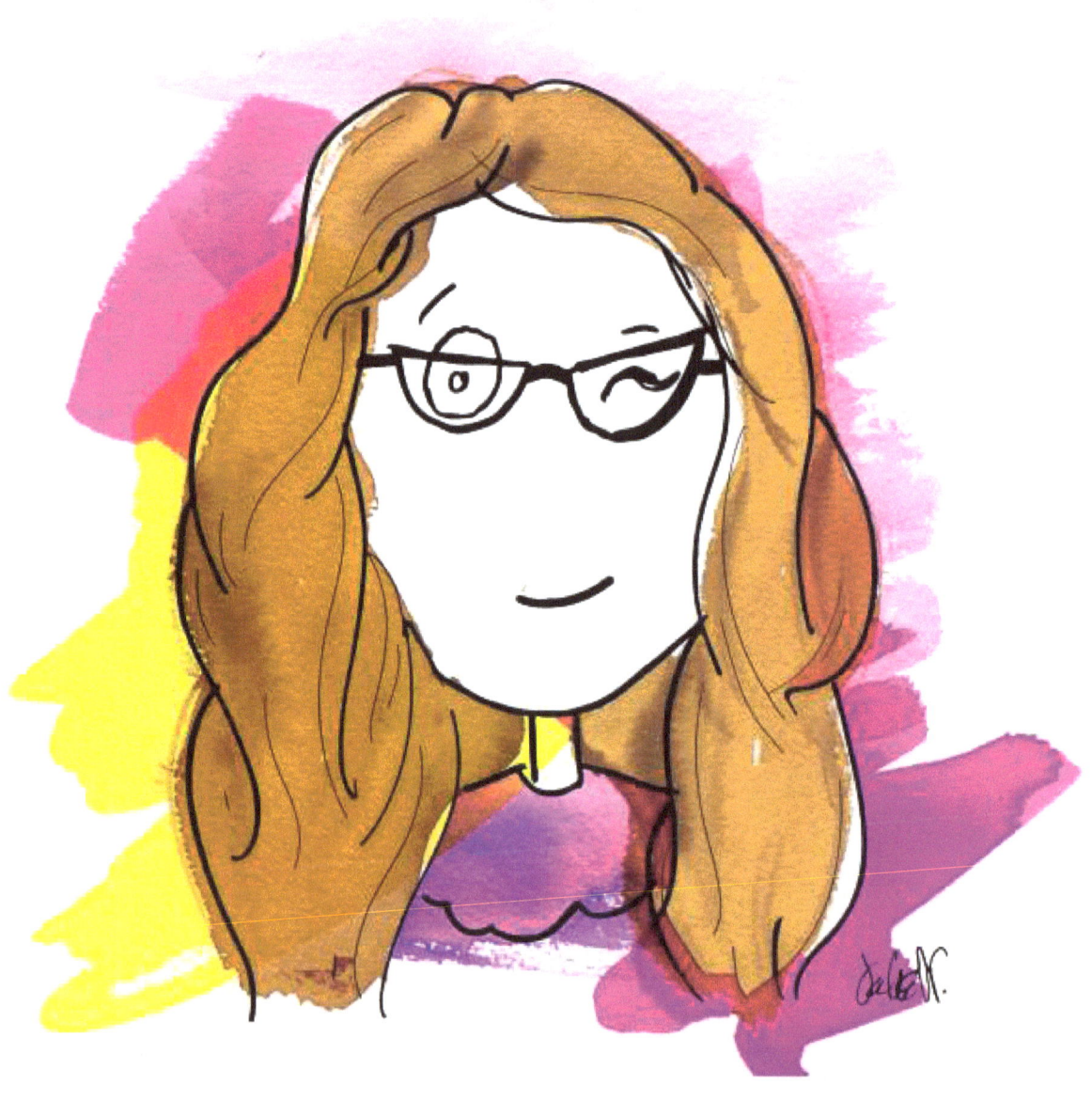

On the board a circle she did draw
"This is like your plate...

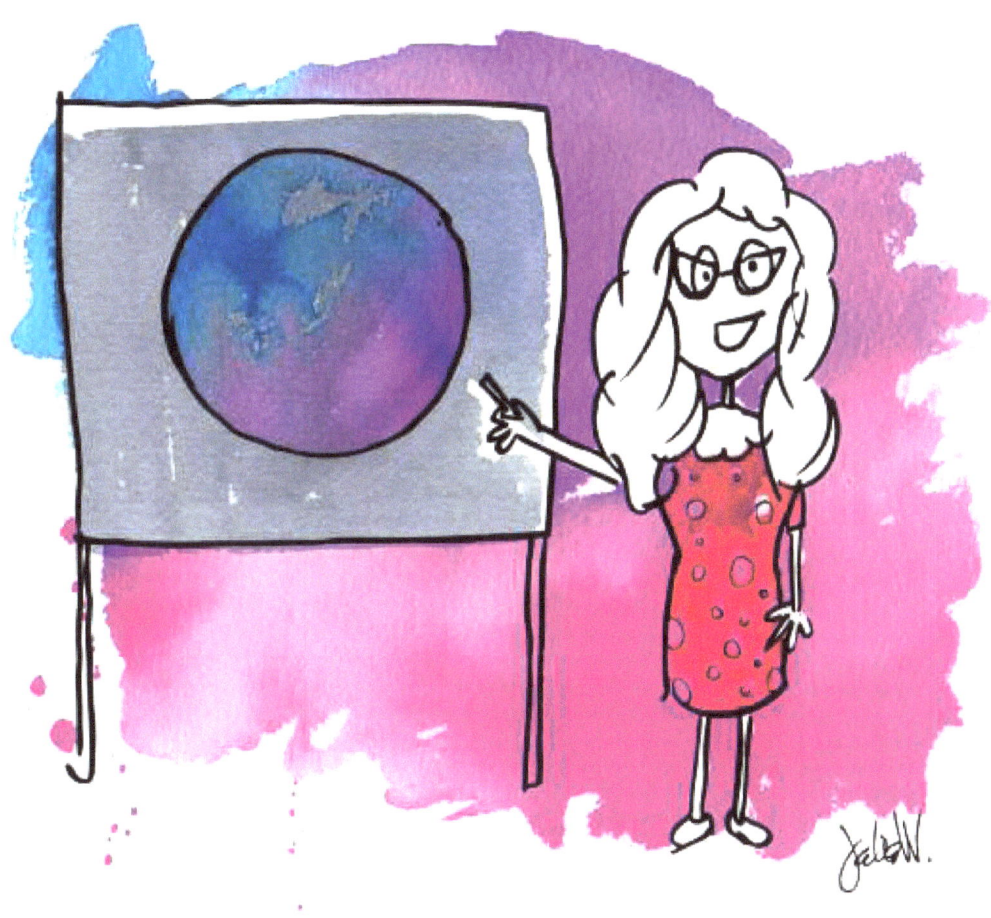

"If you fill it with the Rainbow Foods
You're really gonna feel great."

Red is for strawberries and
red peppers, too,

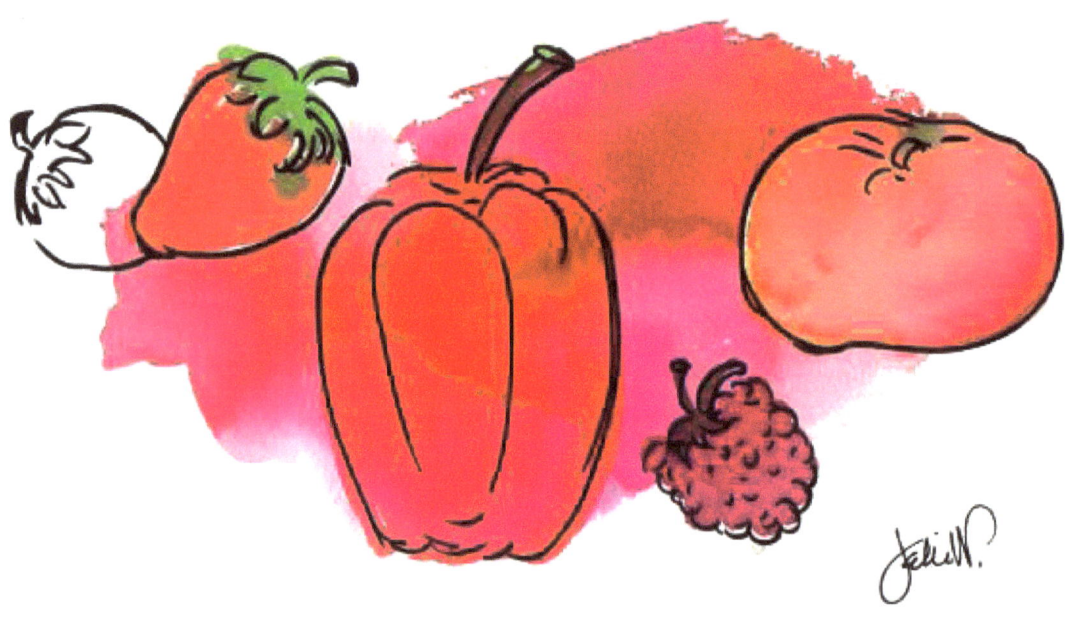

raspberries, tomatoes,
they're all good for you,

Oranges and pumpkins and
tangerines sweet,

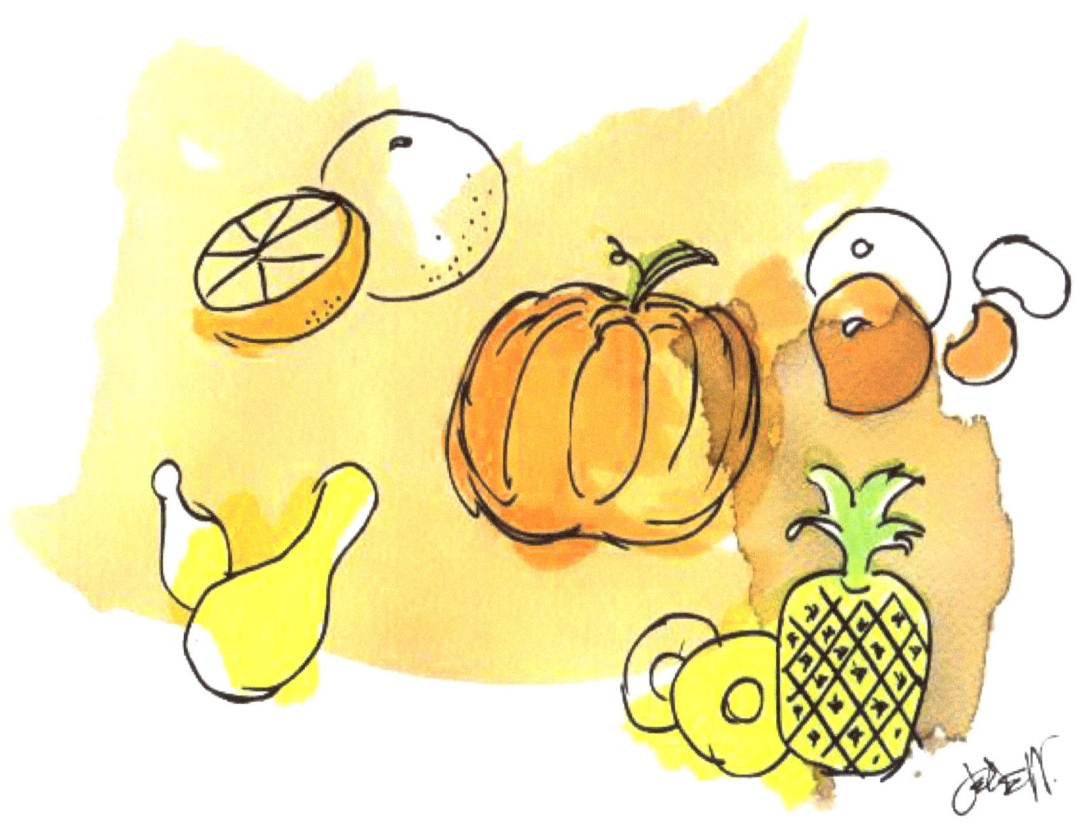

yellow squash and pineapple,
now that's a treat!

Green is for broccoli and
lettuce and beans,

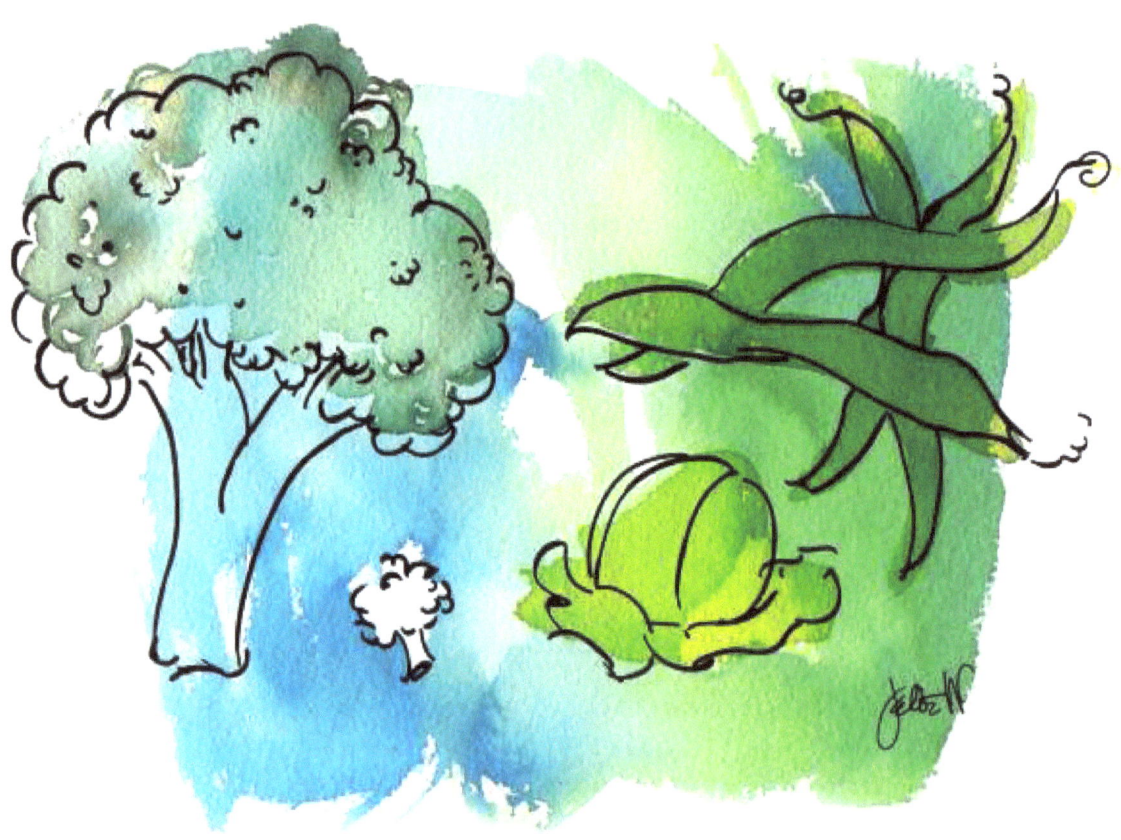

Cabbage and spinach

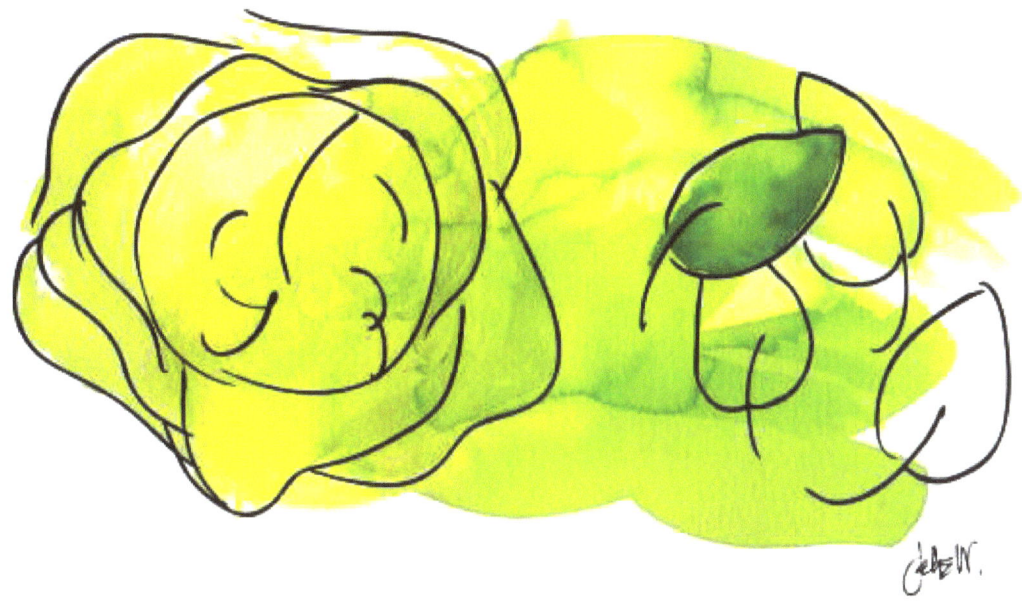

these things are keen.

Blueberries and blackberries

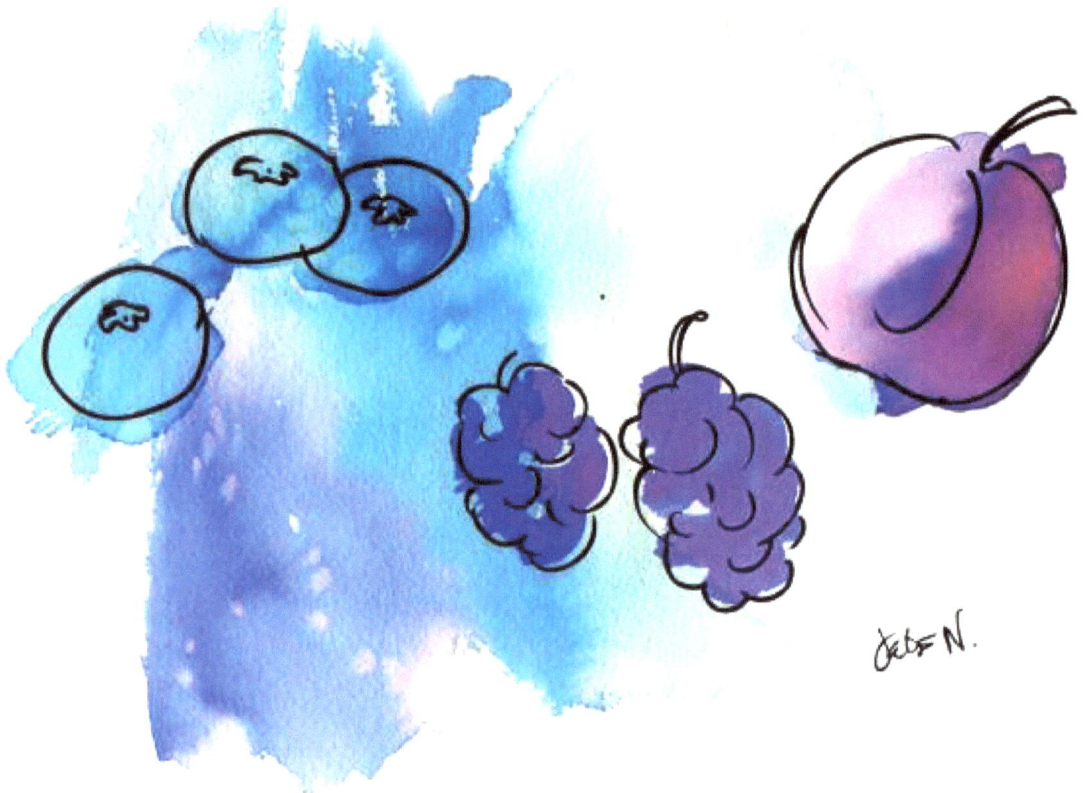

and plums so dark,

With all these good foods
you'll enjoy the Park.

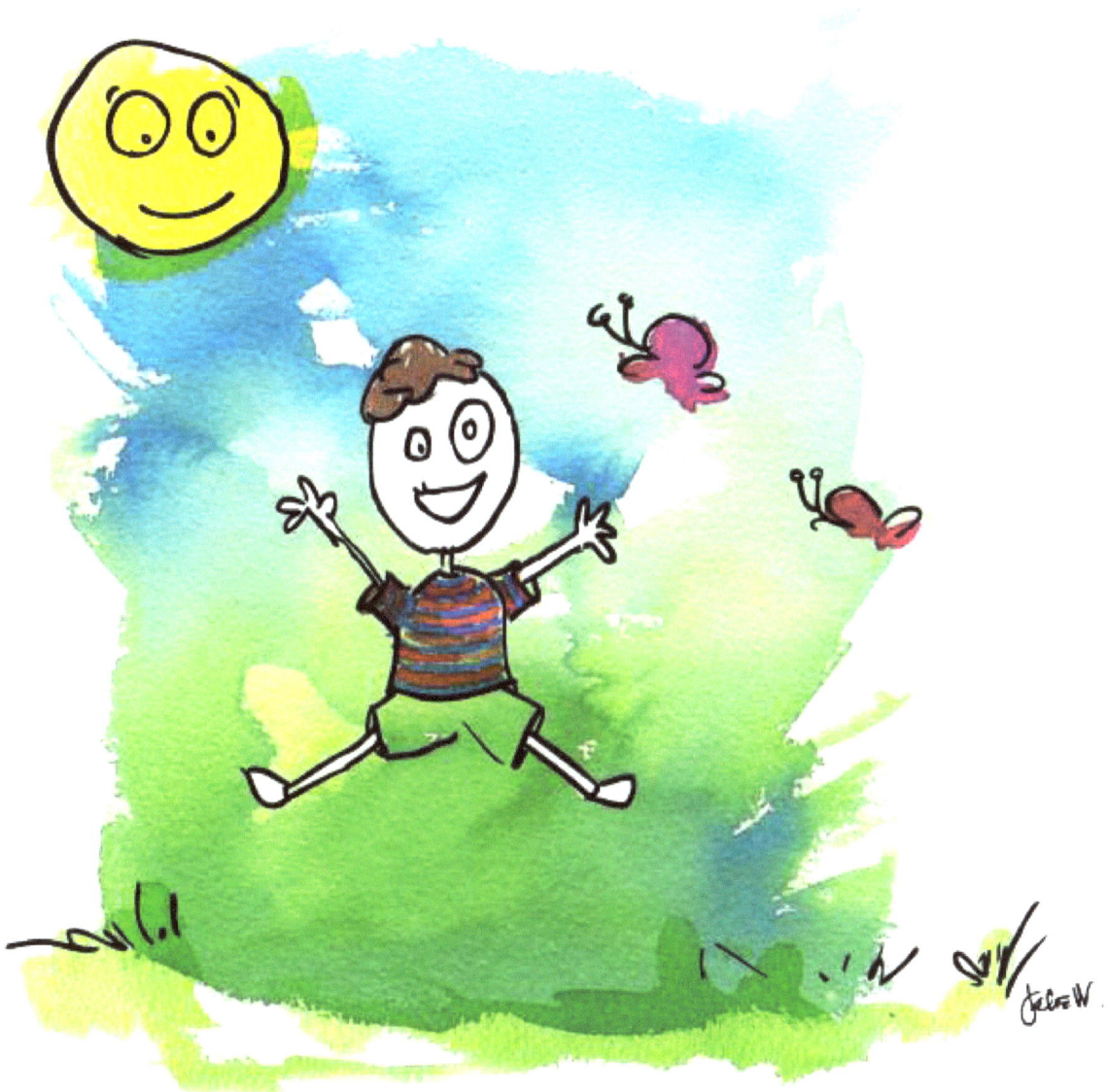

So, remember the colors of
the Rainbow Plate,

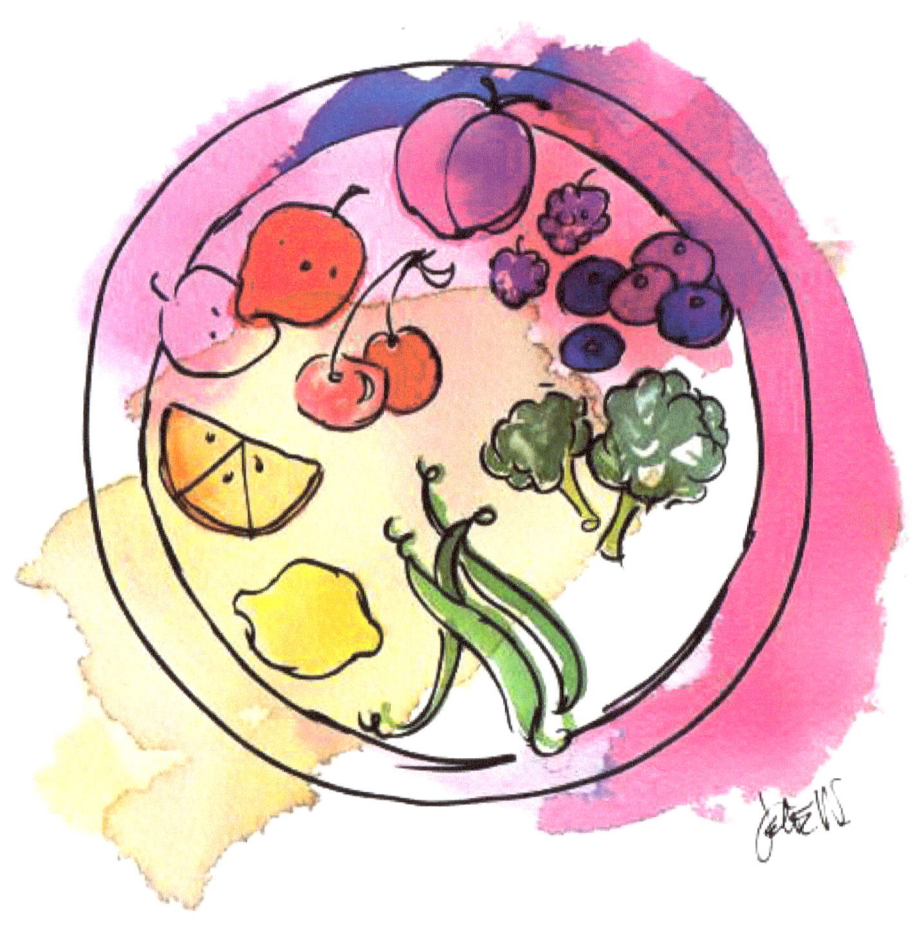

at every meal eat at least three.

And you will be without a doubt -

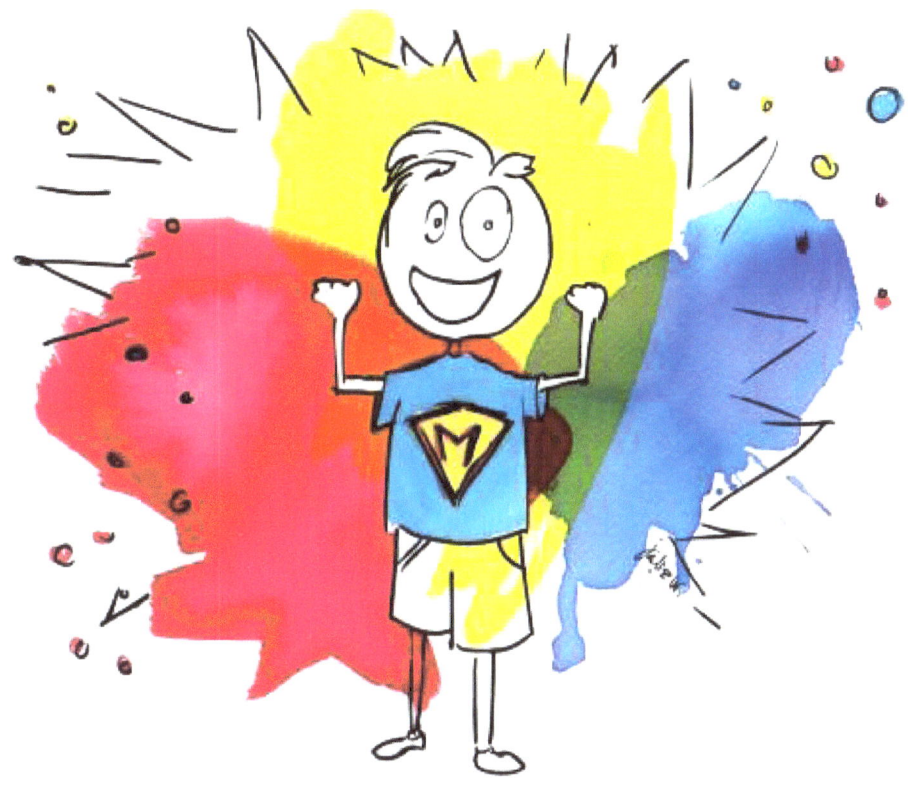

a Super Kid - - the Mighty - Me!

www.ingramcontent.com/pod-product-compliance
Lightning Source LLC
Chambersburg PA
CBHW041526280526
45792CB00004B/1396